HEALTHY EATING AND LIFESTYLE

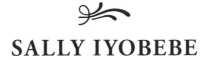

SALLY IYOBEBE

Order this book online at www.trafford.com
or email orders@trafford.com

Most Trafford titles are also available at major online book retailers.

Printed in the United States of America.

ISBN: 978-1-4669-5276-8 (sc)
ISBN: 978-1-4669-5275-1 (e)

Trafford rev. 08/21/2012

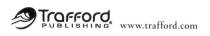 www.trafford.com

North America & international
toll-free: 1 888 232 4444 (USA & Canada)
phone: 250 383 6864 ♦ fax: 812 355 4082

CONTENTS

Apostle Kyle Searcy, Senior Pastor
Fresh Anointing House of Worship

About twenty years ago I began to be awakened to the importance of nutrition. After years of eating any and everything I wanted I began to learn how many of us are digging our graves with our teeth. The old adage is true; we really are what we eat. As one comical pastor puts it, "what goes in the lips will show on the hips." God created so many wonderful healthy foods that will energize and repair our bodies if we would just eat more of them. The body is an amazing creation. When given the right stuff it will function optimally.

In this book Sally Iyobebe masterfully instructs the reader concerning proper eating and nutrition. She shares in great detail the what, why and how of nutrition. If we follow her guidelines our life will be better. This book takes a difficult subject and makes it easy. It is immensely practical. It's scholarly yet simple. It's a how to manual describing how we should live. If you read this book and don't change it will be the greatest waste of time in your life. You must read with a mind to repent where repentance is proper. For you it may truly be a matter of life and death. Read on and Live

ENDORSEMENTS

Rev. Dr. Donatus C. Okafor
President/General Overseer: Divine Touch Ministries Worldwide.

I have known Sister Sally Iyobebe for sometime now. She is a humble, dynamic and an experienced servant of God.

This is a vital subject that must be given a serious attention to if we are to live a scripture fulfilled life.

I recommend it to all Christians and encourage all to read it and listen to the leading of the Holy Spirit for deeper revelation.

DEDICATION

I wish to dedicate this book to the Almighty God for the Grace and courage without which it could not have been a reality.

Also to all the VIRTUOUS WOMEN
(Proverbs 31: 10-31)

ACKNOWLEDGEMENT

I want to give Glory to God the Almighty for the break through regarding this book.

Special thanks to my husband, Mr. Kingsley Iyobebe (The King) for giving me the opportunity to use part of his time to write this book and to use his own time to proofread it.

Special thanks to my Apostle, Apostle Kyle Searcy and Rev. Dr. Donatus Okafor for agreeing to use their time to write the Preface.

I want to acknowledge Mr. Earl Thomas for typesetting this book ready for publication.

Many thanks to my mother, a retired school teacher and a devoted woman of God who taught me how to cook, and to be a hardworking woman, her sweet advice and wonderful prayers.

CHAPTER ONE

What is Nutrition?

Nutrition is the science of crafting food into fuel for the body. Excellent nutrition has several advantages for proper health. The body needs substantial amounts of a definite nutrient and these can be gotten from the following six categories: carbohydrates, proteins, fats, vitamins, minerals, and water. Sugar, starch, and cellulose are all components of carbohydrates. The chemical structures of fats are either saturated or unsaturated. Cholesterol is a fat like substance. Proteins are composed of the severally amino acids. High quality proteins contain sufficient amounts of all essential amino acids while low quality proteins do not. Some minerals are needed in relatively huge amounts. Others are called trace elements because they are needed in barely perceptible amounts. Water too is very important. Each nutrient has the tendency of performing a definite amount of functions in the body and these functions of several nutrients are interrelated. Each type of food has almost the same nutritional content, though they vary in specific values. A combination of a variety of diets helps to ascertain nutritional adequacy.

Nutrition could also be the process whereby food is consumed, nourished, digested and absorbed in to the body for the sustenance of a health and growth.

Importance of Nutrition

1. It provides energy and vibrancy.

Energy is needed for the day to day physical and mental activities. Upon digestion, food eating is broken into smaller molecules such as glucose, amino acids, fats and vitamins. These molecules and nutrients are the elements that provide energy in the body. Carbohydrates eating are broken down into glucose and are stored into the body. Fatty acids brake down fat molecules which become the main source of providing energy to the body. It should be noted, however, that, excess carbohydrates and fat can result in several complications that can lead to obesity and other health diseases.

2. Produces and keeps cells alive and repairs body tissues.

Of the cells present in the body are egg, bones, fat, muscle, brain, nerve and blood cells. All these cells have functions to perform as the body loses cells, it makes new ones. The body tissues are made up of millions of cells. The nutrients that travel through the bloodstream prevent damage, keep cells alive and help in producing new ones.

When amino acids broken down from the consumption of protein food, this aids in building and repairing body tissues.

3. Aids in the Prevention of diseases.

Eating fresh vegetables and fruits daily can help lower blood cholesterol level and prevent heart disease. All fresh fruits and vegetables are nutritious because they are rich in water which is needed to cleanse the system. Fruits especially those that contain bioflavonoid keep the blood from thickening and plugging up the arteries.

4. Necessary during illness and in recuperating.

When in illness or recuperating, it is of importance to eat the right food to maintain or regain the body energy. As therapy and recuperating are painful periods which can affect ones appetite, it is extremely important to eat proper nutrition as to promote faster recovery and health. You should also eat right to prevent infection and other health issues.

5. Assists in the elimination of wastes.

Waste and toxic materials from indigestible food burden your body. It is recommended to eat a healthy diet that contains lots of fresh fruits and vegetables to help cleanse and ease the process of eliminating waste matter.

The body should be taken better care of because it is a means of transportation from and to aid in the actualizations of ones dreams. Sometimes, food supplements and vitamins can be taken as a way of compensating a nutrients deficiency.

CHAPTER TWO

Types of Nutrients

There are five major types of Nutrients:

Carbohydrates

The first class of nutrients come from a wide array of foods such as bread, beans, milk, popcorn, potatoes, cookies, spaghetti, corn, and cherry pie. They also come in a variety of forms. The most common and abundant are sugars, fibers, and starches. The basic building block of a carbohydrate is a sugar molecule, a simple union of carbon, hydrogen, and oxygen. Starches and fibers are essentially chains of sugar molecules. Some contains hundreds of sugars. Some chains are straight, others branch wildly.

Carbohydrates were once grouped into two main categories. Simple carbohydrates included sugars such as fruit sugar (fructose), corn or grape sugar (dextrose or glucose), and table sugar (sucrose). Complex carbohydrates included everything made of three or more linked sugars. Simple sugars were considered bad and complex carbohydrates good.

The digestive system handles all carbohydrates in much the same way and breaks them down or tries to break them down into single sugar molecules, since only these are small enough to cross into the bloodstream. It also converts most digestible carbohydrates into glucose (also known as blood sugar), because cells are designed to use this as a universal energy source.

Fiber is an exception. It is put together in such a way that it can not be broken down into sugar molecules, and so passes through the body undigested.

Carbohydrates serve to provide the body with quick sources of energy. Insufficient amounts of carbohydrates may result in weight loss, fatigue and general lack of energy. A severe deficiency will result in Marasmus and Kwashiorkor.

Proteins

The second class of nutrient consists of proteins. Proteins are large, complex molecules that play many critical roles in the body. They do most of the work in cells and are required for the structure, function, and regulation of the body's tissues and organs. And like carbohydrates, supply energy. The latter is demonstrated in periods of fasting, when the body converts proteins from muscle tissue to energy for use by the body.

Proteins are made up of hundreds or thousands of smaller units called amino acids, which are attached to one another in long chains. There are 20 different types of amino acids that can be combined to make a protein. Complete proteins contain all the amino acids, whereas incomplete proteins lack some of the essential amino acids. Complete proteins are those found in meats. Incomplete proteins are found in vegetables.

Other food sources of complete proteins include animal sources, milk, eggs, cheese, fish, and poultry. Other sources of incomplete proteins are vegetables, fruits, nuts, legumes, peas, beans, and lentils.

Not only are muscles made of proteins, but all body tissues contain some proteins.

Fats

The third class of nutrients which is an important source of calories is fat. Fat is also needed to carry and store essential fat-soluble vitamins, like vitamins A and D. There are two basic types of fat. They are grouped by their chemical structure. Each type of fat is used differently in our bodies and has a different effect on our health.

When we eat a lot of high fat foods, we get a lot of calories. when we ingest too many calories, we may gain weight. Eating too much fat may also increase the risk of getting diseases like cancer, heart disease, high blood pressure or stroke. It is better not to get more than 30% of our calories from fat to reduce our risk of getting these diseases.

Fat is found in many foods. Some of the fat that we eat comes from the fat we add in cooking or spread on breads, vegetables or other foods. A lot of fat is hidden in foods that we eat as snacks, pastries or prepared meals.

We can reduce the amount of fat we eat by cutting down on the fat that we add in cooking or spread on foods. We can eat skim milk and low fat cheeses instead of whole milk and cheese. We can also use less fat, oil, butter, and margarine. Another way to cut down on fat is to drain and trim meats and take the skin off poultry. We can also read labels and compare the amount of fat in foods to make lower fat choices.

Vitamins

The fourth group consists of the vitamins. Fat-soluble vitamins, such as vitamins A, D, E, and K are stored in the liver and disposed as tissues. They must have protein carrier molecules to carry them to their destinations.

Water soluble vitamins such as thiamin, riboflavin, the B complex vitamins, folic acid, and vitamin C are required daily. These vitamins may be lost through improper food preparation. They travel freely through the circulatory and lymphatic systems, to be stored in lean tissues for a month or more. Excess vitamins are excreted by the kidneys.

Vitamin A ensures that the skin and hair are healthy. It also helps to maintain a state of resistance to infection of the eyes, respiratory tract and digestive system. It is required for good eyesight. Food sources of vitamin A are fish liver oil, butter, cream, and dark green and dark yellow vegetables.

Vitamin D is known as the sunshine vitamin and works to help the body to better use calcium and phosphorus. It can be obtained from such food sources as fish liver oils and milk enriched with vitamin D.

Vitamin E has significant functions in relation to human metabolism. It speeds up healing. It can be obtained from foods such as vegetables oils, milk, eggs, meats, cereals, and leafy vegetables.

Vitamin K is essential for clotting of the blood, should a person become wounded or the blood's viscosity very thin. It is found in green, leafy vegetables, liver, soybean, and vegetable oils.

Thiamin maintains healthy nerves and is needed for the metabolism of carbohydrates. It is found in fruits, vegetables, whole grain, and enriched cereal products.

Riboflavin helps keep the skin, mouth and eyes healthy, and helps to maintain resistance to infection. Food sources of riboflavin are milk, meat, whole grain, enriched grain products, fruits, and vegetables.

Niacin increases resistance to infection and prevents pellagra. Sources of niacin include milk, meat, dark green and deep yellow vegetables, and whole grain and enriched grain products.

Ascorbic acid or vitamin C as it is more often called, increases resistance to infections and also keeps teeth and gums in good condition. It can be found in citrus fruits, green and yellow vegetables, milk, and meat.

Insufficient consumption of vitamins may cause severe deficiencies. Deficiencies of niacin can cause pellagra, an illness characterized by diarrhea, dementia, and dermatitis. Lack of vitamin A can result in exophthalmia, an eye disease that can result in blindness. Deficiency of thiamin results in beriberi, or numbness of the feet, legs, arms and muscles, as well as degeneration. Lack of vitamin C will result in scurvy, characterized by loss of weight, sore, bleeding and swollen gums and loss of teeth. Lack of vitamin D causes an illness called ostemalacia, or softening of the bones in the wrists and ankles. Another consequence of insufficient vitamin D is rickets, or bow leggedness, and knocked knees.

Minerals

Minerals are chemical elements, rather than organic compounds, necessary for the health and maintenance of body functions. A key constituent of bones and teeth, calcium is essential for vital metabolic processes such as nerve function, muscle contraction, and blood clotting. Calcium is commonly found in dairy products. A lack of calcium may result in osteomalacia, osteoporosis, rickets, or tetany.

Iron is essential for the transfer of oxygen between body tissues. Hemoglobin carries iron throughout the circulatory system. Iron may be found in eggs, liver, fortified foods such as cereals and white flour, meat, nuts, peas, whole grains, and in green, leafy vegetables. A lack of iron can lead to anemia and an increased susceptibility to infections.

Magnesium is essential for healthy bones and aids in the formation of compounds needed for energy conversion. Magnesium is found in milk, most fruits, pulses, and leafy, green vegetables. A lack of magnesium may lead to anemia, demineralization of bones, nerve disorders, respiratory problems, weakness, and weight loss.

As the main base ion of intercellular fluid, sodium maintains the pH balance of the body and is necessary to maintain the electrical potentials of the nervous system and the functioning of muscle and nerve tissues. Sodium is found in processed bakery products, table salt and in processed foods such as canned goods and cured products. Insufficient sodium in the diet may lead to low blood pressure general muscle weakness or paralysis, mild fever, and respiratory problems. Excess sodium, on the other hand, may lead to dehydration and hypertension.

Other minerals needed in trace amounts include chromium, copper, manganese, selenium, sulphur, and zinc.

CHAPTER THREE

What the Bible says about our body

The Bible tells us our body is the temple of the Lord. And that means that as a temple, it should be nurtured and cared for. Having a healthy body improves the quality of life for our selves, and for the people around us. You can be a more powerful blessing to others when you are energetic and healthy.

In his book "Overcoming Lust of the Flesh", Apostle Kyle Searcy Wrote:

"Know ye not that your body is the temple of the Holy Ghost which is in you, which ye have of God, and ye are not your own"? For ye are bought with a price: therefore glorify God in your body, and in your spirit, which are God's" (1 Corinthians 6:19-20). He said that should settle the fact. That our bodies belong to God. So we should do what pleases God and not what pleases us. Paul tells us to glorify God in our body, as well as our spirit. Princess of Zion Center, Inc. wants to create the awareness through seminars, evangelism, talk shows, backyard garden, and vocational education on how we should treat our bodies as the temple of God through proper nutrition by growing and cooking our own food.

1. Health and Healing

Disease is a curse and our Lord Jesus Christ has redeemed us from the curse on the cross of Calvary. Apostle Kyle Searcy again in one of his sermons tells us to discover the fullness of our redemption and how salvation frees us not only from sin and sickness but from the spirit of darkness. He said Jesus Christ has liberated us from all of our infirmities by taking away all our sins, diseases, and our troubles. (Matthew 8:17). And that Jesus Christ did not only take away our sins, He also took away our diseases when He was on that Cross. Apostle Kyle has this vexation of Christian after receiving salvation falls back into the veils of the enemy's/ world. He said a Christian after receiving salvation may continue to lure after wards but he does not have to. He said sin does not have to Lord over us unless and except we allow it to happen. (Romans. 6: 14) We have been redeemed from sin and sickness, the price has been paid for our healing. The Lord Jesus Christ has given us the weapon to bind, reject, denounce and cast out freely all kinds of sicknesses and diseases. That is to say our faith has to be at the level of the knowledge of God's word. And then we will begin to operate in divine health.

As one accepts the fact that as surely as Jesus Christ died on the Cross was mainly to bare our sins, then we will have to understand that He has also taken away our pains, diseases, sufferings, and weakness, then we will realize the days of our glory has come.

If you are engrossed in the Word of God it will destroy all the grips of Satan in our lives pertaining to the area of physical suffering. When one believes and has faith, he/she is automatically sets free from Christ dominion when one comes to terms that his/her healing has already been bought by our Lord Jesus Christ on the Cross. The truth is He has taken away our—grieves, pains, sickness, weakness and our sorrows. Upon all we still have disregard for Him. He was wounded for our transgressions, he was bruised for our iniquities: the chastisement of our peace was upon him; and with his stripes we are healed" (Isaiah 53:4-5).

Jesus bore sin and sickness in order for us to be set free. As sin is the manifestation of spiritual death in the heart of man, sickness is the manifestation of spiritual death in the body of man.

Not only did Jesus pay the price for the new birth of our spirit and the healing of our body, He also bore the chastisement of our peace. Satan has no right to torment us physically, mentally and spiritually. We have been redeemed from fear, frustration and confusion, mental anxiety, depression, aggression, spiritual oppression, shame, demonic padlock/chains, occult and many more that will want to keep us from enjoying our Godly peace. We do not need any medication or soothsayer to keep us abreast. Jesus has paid the price for us. All we need to do is just run to Him with any problem and He is just willing to accept us. Let us not allow Satan to come in between us and our peace of mind.

2.   Total Redemption

Jesus came to destroy all the works of the devil (1 John 3:8). He did not destroy sin only to leave sickness in dominion. Partial redemption from Satan's power would not have pleased God nor would it have fulfilled His plan for His family.

He redeemed the whole man righteousness for his nature, peace for his mind and healing for his body. Redemption left nothing in force that came upon man because of sin. Jesus completely destroyed the works of the devil in the lives of men.

First Corinthians 6:20 says, "For ye are bought with a price." A great price! "Therefore glorify God in your body, and in your spirit, which are God's." There should not be any sickness in the Body of Christ. When one who is sick comes into our midst, the healing power of God should flow so that he receives healing.

In the book of Leviticus, Israel used a scapegoat. The priest laid hands on a real goat, put the sins of the people on him and sent him to the wilderness totally away from the people. That's what Jesus did with our sickness and disease. He bore them away from us.

So let us stand up in the Name of Jesus and command sickness and disease to go away from us. We should refuse to allow any kind of sickness in our body. We should cast it out of our very presence, command sickness or diseases to depart from our bodies and that of our families.

3. Salvation.

What does it mean to be saved? How do you know when you have been saved? And how do you know if you are born again?

What is salvation?

Salvation is one of the promises of God to all believers: to be given the gift of eternal life. To be "saved" in the full sense of the word means to have received eternal life. The word salvation is also used to describe the process we go through before we can receive eternal life. "Saved" refers to redemption, one of the steps in the process of salvation. Here are two of many verses about eternal life:

For God so loved the world, that he gave his only begotten Son, that whosoever believeth in him should not perish, but have everlasting life. (John 3:16)

For the wages of sin is death; but the gift of God is eternal life through Jesus Christ our Lord. (Romans 6:23)

Salvation is not just the new birth of our spirit. It is also peace of mind and healing for the body. Salvation denotes "deliverance, preservation; material and temporal deliverance from danger and apprehension."

Mark 16:15-16 says, "Go ye into the entire world, and preach the gospel to every creature. He that believeth and is baptized shall be saved; but he that believeth not shall be damned." The gospel is the good news of what Jesus did in His substitution sacrifice at the cross.

"By whose stripes ye were healed" is not a promise. It is a fact. It has already taken place. Jesus bore sickness away from us, and by His stripes we were healed.

There is no sin so great that Jesus' sacrifice at Calvary will not cancel it and wipe it away as though sin had never been. The power of God cleanses and changes one who partakes of the gift of salvation until there is no trace of the old man or his sins. When we are born again, we become a new man, a new creature. Our new spirit is created in the righteousness of God.

There is no disease so devastating to the human body that the same sacrifice at Calvary will not cancel it and wipe it away and heal that body as though sickness had never been.

The gospel is the good news of what Jesus did for every person by sacrificing His life at the cross for us. He bore our sins, so we do not have to bear them. Now we can be forgiven. He did that for every sinner by bearing our diseases, so that we do not have to bear them any longer. We can be healed right away. He did that for every sick person and every sufferer.

That is why the gospel is called good news because of what Jesus Christ did for us mankind.

Jesus commanded that this good news be preached to every creature because everyone who hears it and believes it will be saved and healed.

As the Body of Christ, we do not have to tolerate sickness any longer. Jesus paid the price for our redemption from the curse of the law. That is even though Jesus bore our sins and sickness, and we have received freedom, we still have to avoid eating what we know is not healthy for the body as these things can cause sin and diseases to enter our body. Let us not forget that all this has to be by the blood of our Lord Jesus Christ.

CHAPTER FOUR

You are what you eat

We have all heard the old adage 'you are what you eat', but have never stopped to think exactly how true that is? Simply put, healthy eating is the key to wellbeing. We all have up to 100 trillion cells in our bodies, each one demanding a constant supply of daily nutrients in order to function optimally. Food affects all of these cells, and by extension, every aspect of our being: mood, energy levels, food cravings, thinking capacity, sex drive, sleeping habits and general health. If you feed your body junk and convenience foods it'll simply lay down fat, lower your energy, and even diminish your brain power.

According to The CDC-Chronic Disease-Obesity-At a Glance, "more than one third of U.S. adults, more than 72 million people, and 16% of U.S. children are obese. Since 1980, obesity rates for adults have doubled and rates for children have tripled. Obesity rates among all groups in society, irrespective of age, sex, race, ethnicity, socioeconomic status, educational level, or geographic region, have increased remarkably."

Health Consequences of Obesity

Obesity has physical, psychological, and social consequences in adults and children. Children and adolescents are developing obesity-related diseases, such as type 2 diabetes, that were once seen only in adults. Obese children are more likely to have risk factors for cardiovascular disease, including high cholesterol levels, high blood pressure, and abnormal glucose tolerance. One study of 5- to 17-year-olds found that 70% of obese children had at least one risk factor for cardiovascular disease and 39% of obese children had at least two risk factors.

Few doubt that overweight people, women in particular are often treated differently than slimmer folks. That type of treatment may be troubling to the point of being stressful. This is a struggle that, causes women to feel embarrassed.

Four themes usually become apparent to these women.

1. struggling to fit in,
2. Feeling not quite human,
3. Being dismissed, and
4. Refusing to give up.

This book is a wake up call and offers some advice. Whether you are struggling with your weight, feeling like you have no energy, suffering from stress, have specific health problems, or just want to feel more alive, this is the time to rethink

Some tips about excellent eating

1. Avoid sugar—found in cakes, biscuits, confectionary, chocolate, candy, desserts, soft drinks and many other foods.

2. Use whole grains rather than refined carbohydrates—white bread, white flour, white pastry, white pasta and white rice should be replaced with brown rice, quinoa, millet, oats, barley, rye, buckwheat and red rice.

3. Avoid artificial additives—these may be sweeteners, preservatives, colorings or flavorings.

4. Avoid stimulants—caffeine, alcohol, nicotine and other recreational drugs.

5. Eat vegetables or salads with lunch and dinner—Variety is important, so experiment with those that you don't normally eat.

6. Include some sources of essential fats every day—these include oily fish (such as salmon, mackerel, sardines, herrings and trout), pumpkin seeds, sunflower seeds, sesame seeds, linseeds/flaxseeds, hemp seeds, walnuts and avocadoes. Avoid processed fats such as low fat spreads and margarines.

7. Have at least 2 vegetarian days each week. Good vegetarian proteins include chickpeas, lentils, mung beans, brocolli, beans, butter beans, aduki beans, tofu, tempeh, quinoa, amaranth, nuts and seeds.

8. Avoid processed meats—ham, salami, chorizo, hot dogs, bacon and any smoked or cured meats. These all contain nitrates that have been linked to stomach cancer and are high in saturated fats and salt which are linked to cardiovascular disease.

9. Cook from scratch whenever possible—this means buying whole, natural ingredients and cooking or preparing them yourself. Avoid processed and packaged foods as much as possible.

10. Buy locally grown, organically produced, seasonal produce where possible—check out farmer's markets, farm shops and pick-your-own farms for the freshest produce.

Gluttony and Self Control

"Excess." Derived from the Latin glutton, meaning to gulp down or swallow. Gluttony (Latin, gula) is the over indulgence and over consumption of anything to the point of waste. In the Christian religions, it is considered a sin because of the excessive desire for food, or its withholding from the needy.

Depending on the culture, it can be seen as either a vice or a sign of status. Where food is relatively scarce, being able to eat well might be something to take pride in. But in an area where food is routinely plentiful, it may be considered a sign of self-control to resist the temptation to over-indulge.

Medieval church leaders (e.g., Thomas Aquinas) took a more expansive view of gluttony, arguing that it could also include an obsessive anticipation of meals, and the constant eating of delicacies and excessively costly foods. Aquinas went so far as to prepare a list of six ways to commit gluttony, including:

Praepropere—eating too soon.

Laute—eating too expensively.

Nimis—eating too much.

Ardenter-eating too eagerly (burningly).

Studiose—eating too daintily (keenly).

Forente—eating wildly (boringly).

CHAPTER FIVE

Fasting

Fasting is the practice of denying oneself food, beverages or both in order to concentrate on a relationship with God and the pursuit of a state of unity with Him, or in the pursuit of an intention that is desired from God. Removing the chore of eating from a daily schedule frees up time to be spent on spiritual pursuits, such as reading Holy Scriptures or praying in personal communication with God. Fasting allows one to concentrate and meditate on the precepts of the Lord, to meditate on his word for a period of time. This time period can be short or long. Not only do people fast for different time periods, but they also fast for different reasons.

Many think that fasting is only about food, but it can also mean abstaining from favorite activities such as sex, watching television or shopping.

Fasting has been around since the time of the Biblical patriarchs 4,000 years ago and before. Fasting was practiced by adherents in both the Old and New Testaments. For instance, Moses fasted for two recorded forty day periods. Jesus fasted 40 days and reminded his followers to fast. "When you fast," not "if you fast." The Bible is replete with instances of the spiritual leaders—for example Onias the High Priest of the Israelites, calling for a time of national prayer and fasting. The prophets would often don sackcloth and ashes in order to fast and pray before the Lord.

Time Frame

Fasts can be carried out for varying periods. Some people like to fast from sun up to sun down so that they finish the fast with the evening meal. Yom Kippur in the Jewish calendar is a total 24-hour fast, during which nothing at all is eaten or drunk and the day is spent in the synagogue praying and worshipping God. Of course there are the 40 day fasts of Jesus and Moses mentioned previously, and many churches practice the three day and seven day dry fast, which culminates with a time of fellowship and breaking of bread. It is not wise to have a huge meal to break the fast, especially after a longer fast.

Considerations.

To prepare for this special communion with God, it is important that the person engaging in the fast should examine their own conscience and heart to clear themselves of any lingering sins. Scripture tells us that God requires his people to repent of sins before he will hear their prayers. Psalm 66:16-20 tells us, "Come and hear, all of you who reverence the Lord, and I will tell you what he did for me: For I cried to him for help, with praises ready on my tongue. He would not have listened if I had not confessed my sins. But he listened. He heard my prayer. He paid attention to it. Blessed be God who did not turn away when I was praying, and did not refuse me his kindness and love."

Warning

Although fasting is an important part of the spiritual realm, it has its roots in the physical. Before fasting there should be some basic preparations. When fasting for an extended period, say a week, it is helpful to prepare ones self by eating smaller meals before you totally cease eating altogether.

Do not have a huge meal before you begin, thinking that this will last you over the fast. Instead you should cut down on large meals and get your stomach used to smaller and smaller meals. Some nutritionists suggest eating only uncooked foods before starting a fast. Others also recommend cutting caffeine and sugar to ease hunger or discomfort at the early stages of the fast.

Effects of fasting

Although fasting will be a great blessing if done in the Spirit of humility, it can not always be done by everyone. Those people who do fast may experience mental and physical discomforts. There are inner doubts that may arise, especially if you have a particular liking for some delicacy that you have denied yourself. Personally I have found taking Jesus' words in Matthew 4:3 to heart "Man does not live by bread alone, but by every word that comes from the mouth of God", to be very helpful. Whenever I have pangs of hunger or regret for food, while fasting, I pick up the Bible and read his Word until the craving has passed.

Time Frame

Most people fast for only short periods of time such as one day, or up to a week. Some fasts can last as long as a month, but such a fast will generally be limited to choice foods or activities. The most extreme fasts are the political fasts, which can last until the subject becomes very ill, or until they die if the reason they are fasting is not resolved.

Type of fasting

There are several different types of fasting.

Religious fasting: Each religious group has different rules regarding fasting. Christians usually refer to the Book of Isaiah, which refers to afflicting the soul and abstaining from flesh related needs in an effort to purify oneself. For a partial fast that will go on for a long period, the book of Daniel 8-16 can be demonstrated as a good guideline.

Medical fasting: The word fasting in medical terms means the state of the body after a meal has been digested. If a person has not eaten for 8 to 12 hours, then he or she is in a fast state. The fast state allows doctors to get true results on diagnostic tests and it is also wise to have no food in the body during operations.

Political fasting: Fasting is used by people to protest or to bring awareness to an important cause. Hunger strikes are a non violent way of bringing attention to causes.

Fasting for diet: The type of fasting is not recommended, but it is fasting often used as a means to lose weight quickly or to start a diet. While most people lose weight on fasts, they often gain it back just as quickly and damage the body in the process.

Significance of fasting.

The significance of religious fasting is to deprive yourself or your body in an offer of sacrifice in preparation for prayer. Medical fasting is necessary if you are having a medical procedure or tests, as doctors may need your stomach and bowels empty before a procedure or for your blood sugar and over levels to be controlled. A person who fasts publicly for political reasons puts themselves in physical danger for the good of others. The significance of a diet fast could be to give our body and mind a jump start in losing weight before a prolonged diet.

CHAPTER SIX

Eat your way to excellent health

The foods we eat and the lifestyle choices we make play a major role in our health. Healthy choices can:

1. Reduce your risk for developing chronic diseases. High blood pressure, diabetes, heart disease, and some cancers are related to diet and food choices.
2. Control symptoms of medical conditions. High blood pressure, high blood sugar, and high cholesterol may be improved by diet and food choices

Gaining or losing weight is related to diet and exercise. If you take in more calories than your body needs, you are likely to gain weight. To maintain your weight at a healthy level, you must eat fewer calories; increase your exercise, or both. Good reasons for maintaining a healthy weight are the health benefits.

Obesity increases the risk of:

* Cancers of the colon, breast, prostate, and esophagus.
* Heart disease.
* Diabetes.

* High blood pressure.
* Other long-term diseases such as arthritis, gallbladder disease, and asthma.

Control Your Food Portion

Too many calories from any food can result in weight gain. To avoid weight gain, it is essential to control the portions of food you eat.

Understand Food Labels

* Reading and understanding food labels will help you make wise food choices

* Physical Activity:

Being physically active is part of a healthy lifestyle. You can at least do 30-45 minutes of a moderate exercise on weekly basis. This can help you maintain cardiovascular fitness. By so doing it, this will enable you to burn about 200 or more calories a day and about 1000 calories a week.

To be able to reduce or stay at your current weight, you can do about 60 to 120 minutes of moderate to vigorous walking or activities each day of the week. The Gym is not the only place to exercise.

* When in a building that has an elevator, use the stair cases instead of the elevator. Getting off of the bus or subway early and take a walk home.
* Walk to work, class, store, park or the neighbor hood.
* You can also go for a brisk walk or jogging.

* Get your self busy with house hold chores such as vacuuming, mopping, dusting, washing dishes and doing laundry.

  Go swimming with family and friends

* Cycling, Dancing, Gardening, basket ball, Soccer, volley ball, cleaning the yard and raking the leaves and grass are part of healthy exercise.

Water, as the greatest healer

No matter what the specific health or fitness goal, one cannot achieve the maximum benefit from any health program without drinking the right kind of water in the proper amount. All experts agree, that next to the air we breathe, water is the most important thing we will ever put in our bodies. It is surprising that so much time and money is being spent on supplements, organic foods and natural remedies (some of which are very subtle and delicate) but little attention is given to the quality and effect of the water with which those items are taken.

Every function inside the body is regulated by and depends on water. Water must be available to carry vital elements, oxygen, hormones, and chemical messengers to all parts of the body. Without sufficient water to wet all parts equally, some more remote parts of the body will not receive the vital elements that water supplies.

Water is also needed to carry toxic waste away from the cells. In fact, there are at least 50 reasons why the body needs sufficient water on a regular, everyday basis. Without sufficient water to constantly wet all parts, your body's drought management system kicks into action. The histamine directed chemical messenger systems are activated to arrange a new, lower quota of water for the drought stricken areas. When histamine and its subordinate "drought managers" come across pain sensing nerves, they cause pain. This is why dehydration produces pain as its first alarm signal. If the dehydration persists and is not corrected naturally with water, it becomes symptom producing and, in time, develops into a disease condition. This is why people who take antacids to silence their bodies' thirst pain become more vulnerable and eventually develop other serious complications of dehydration.

CHAPTER SEVEN

Understanding Vitamins and Mineral Supplements

Vitamins are organic components that are necessary for human life and health. Vitamins cannot be manufactured in the body (vitamin B12 is an exception) and so must be obtained from diet.

Minerals are inorganic ions (metals) that are also necessary for the life and health.

Minerals are not manufactured in the body and so must be obtained from diet.

Trace minerals which are minerals necessary to the body in extremely small, or trace amounts.

Accessory nutrients are substances that are not absolutely necessary for life and health. They that participate with vitamins and minerals in numerous biochemical reactions.

Taking vitamins is a wise health and preventive measure. Deficiencies of vitamins and minerals cause many diseases. Adding vitamins and minerals, in supplemental form is an inexpensive "insurance policy" against some of the worst diseases of modern times.

A deficiency of antioxidant vitamins and minerals (especially beta carotene, vitamins C and E, and selenium) is associated with higher incidence of cancers of the colon, breast, prostate, mouth, lungs and skin.

A mineral deficiency, especially magnesium and potassium but also calcium, is associated with high blood pressure.

Deficiencies of vitamins E.C. B6, B12, folic acid (a B vitamin), and bioflavonoid are associated with cardiovascular disease. The connection between vitamin E and heart health is so well established that conventional medical cardiologists are instructed to recommend vitamin E to their patients.

Healthy bones, and the prevention of osteoporosis, depend on sufficient levels of minerals, including calcium, magnesium, boron, zinc, copper, B vitamins and vitamin D.

The Sacredness of Food and Eating

This piece was written by Mariel Hemingway, that we all have a relationship to food that is at once joyous and infuriating. Food is a basic essential; we can not get away from it. We have to eat to survive and thrive. Yet it appears, that we have turned desperate around food, by over indulging. We love to eat because we love the feeling that food gives us. It is nurturing, it is grounding. Often, that feeling is a replacement for our sense of well being and love. By nature, humans want more love that's all anybody really wants. So we turn to food to get a sense of self. It's easier that way, because it has no person attached to it, judging us or finding reasons we should not be loved.

So we eat more, because if love is what we desire, we certainly want more of it. We anthropomorphize food, making it our friend, our lover, our partner, our therapist. This takes away the need to look at the deeper issues of why we feel unloved.

Food as a celebratory, that expressive aspect of our life!

Food is such a beautiful part of our lives. I want to invite people and myself to gracefully find a way to turn food into a valued ceremony that enhances our lives on every level. Instead of making food a person, I would like to make food another essence of myself. Food becomes that which expresses my delicacy as a woman and as a being that cares for her.

When food is overindulged in, it takes on qualities of a master and slave. Food becomes the master and the eater becomes its slave. With that, there comes the constant need to please. You become split within yourself. Instead of being true to your essence and your nature, you serve your outer self, the one ruled by the food. If food can come down from the realm of regal master and become our inner essence, everyone benefits. We slow down and eat with conscious awareness of how we chew, how we set a table, what we prepare for the enhancement of our essence.

If food becomes our artistic expression, then we all become very careful in the implementation of our gift. Our making of nourishment becomes the act with which we create something that, like a sand mandala that gets blown out of existence by the wind, is not permanently in sight but is constant in our being. Still, the energy that was put into the food stays with us and moves into our cells, into our sense of self. It becomes the essence of us. It can be healing when we have made it from love instead of using it as the outer expression of a love that is hollow and perhaps not real love at all.

We should focus more on where our food comes from

Real food is like real love; it is born of the earth. It grows like some kind of miracle that we have come to take for granted. Yet the journey we are on right now is to remember where our food has come from, the journey that it has taken from field to plate.

This is not just any kind of stuff! This is awareness of life and how we inhabit the planet. This is about all people becoming themselves deeply, caring for their world by caring for themselves.

To some extent, we make food and try new recipes to satisfy the needs of our bodies and families, and sometimes to impress the outside world. But we can also see it as developing our inner world, using the deliberate act of choosing and cooking food as a very basic practice of becoming more authentic. When we step back, become quiet, and consider that food may come from something greater than ourselves, however we want to picture that, whether as Nature, Spirit, Source, Gaia, or God, our awareness shifts. Food consciousness, I believe, is a foundation of our spiritual life.

Throughout history, in all sacred places, the ritual of food has a profound place in the connection to the spirit. Whether in the preparation, the sacrament, the blessing, the intent, or the symbolism, cooking is understood to be a ritual of connection and devotion. Done consciously, it becomes sacred to the development of your sense of self and your connection to your bigger self, that part of you that is already perfect.

Care for your inner environment by being aware of your participation in the outer environment, that place the sustenance comes from, and you will feel a deeper connection to yourself as a unique expression of the divine.